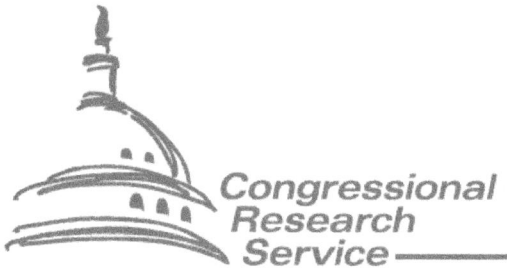

Congressional Research Service

Private Health Insurance Market Reforms in the Patient Protection and Affordable Care Act (ACA)

Annie L. Mach
Analyst in Health Care Financing

Bernadette Fernandez
Specialist in Health Care Financing

April 16, 2012

Congressional Research Service
7-5700
www.crs.gov
R42069

CRS Report for Congress
Prepared for Members and Committees of Congress

Summary

The private health insurance provisions in the Patient Protection and Affordable Care Act (P.L. 111-148, ACA, as amended) include market reforms that impose requirements on private health insurance plans. Such reforms relate to the offer, issuance, generosity, and pricing of health plans, among other requirements.

ACA's market reforms largely focus on the individual and small group health insurance markets, and in this report the reforms have been grouped by effective dates: "immediate" market reforms that become effective *prior* to the full implementation date of ACA, and reforms that become effective *on* the full implementation date (January 1, 2014).

ACA requires implementation of a number of reforms prior to its full implementation date (i.e., prior to plan years beginning on or after January 1, 2014). "Immediate" reforms include a process to review unreasonable rate increases; an Internet portal to assist consumers in identifying coverage options; prohibition on lifetime limits and restriction of annual limits; the prohibition on rescissions; coverage of preventive health services with no cost-sharing; extension of dependent coverage; prohibition of discrimination based on salary; standards related to medical loss ratios and rebates to plan participants; appeals process; coverage of preexisting health conditions for children; patient protections; uniform explanation of coverage documents; and reporting requirements regarding quality of care.

Market reforms effective beginning in 2014 include nondiscrimination based on health status; guaranteed issue and guaranteed renewability; coverage of preexisting health conditions (regardless of age); nondiscrimination regarding clinical trial participation; rating restrictions; waiting period limitation; and nondiscrimination regarding health care providers.

This report provides background information about the private health insurance market, including market segments and regulation. It describes each ACA market reform and notes any major implementation activity that has occurred (e.g., issuance of final rule from a department such as Health and Human Services). The appendices of the report provide additional information about the status of regulations relating to each reform and how the reforms apply to the different market segments and health plans.

Contents

Tables

Appendixes

Contacts

T he Patient Protection and Affordable Care Act (P.L. 111-148, ACA,[1] as amended) includes reforms of the health insurance market that impose requirements on private health insurance plans.[2] Such reforms relate to the offer, issuance, generosity, and pricing of health plans, among other requirements. Certain reforms also require the participation of public agencies and officials, such as the Secretary of Health and Human Services (hereinafter, the Secretary), in order to facilitate administrative or operational functions.

This report provides background information about the private health insurance market, including market segments and regulation. It describes each ACA market reform and notes any major implementation activity that has occurred (e.g., issuance of final rule from a Department such as Health and Human Services). The appendices of the report provide additional information about the status of regulations relating to each reform and how the reforms apply to the different market segments and health plans.

Background

Health Insurance Markets

The private health insurance market is often characterized as having three segments—the large group, small group, and individual markets. Insurance sold in the large and small group markets refers to health plans offered through a plan sponsor, typically an employer.[3] Large groups generally have more than 50 workers. Small groups generally refer to firms with 50 or fewer workers. However, beginning in 2016, ACA will define small groups as employers with 100 or fewer workers, and large groups as employers with more than 100 workers. The individual (nongroup) market refers to insurance policies offered to individuals and families buying insurance on their own (i.e., not through a plan sponsor).

State and Federal Regulation

States are the primary regulators of the business of health insurance, as codified by the 1945 McCarran-Ferguson Act (15 U.S.C. §§1011 *et seq.*). Each state has a large, unique set of rules that apply to state-licensed insurance carriers and the plans they offer.[4] Such rules are broad in scope and address a variety of issues, such as the legal structure and organization of insurance issuers (e.g., licensing requirements), business practices (e.g., marketing rules), market conduct

---

[1] Previous CRS reports on the Patient Protection and Affordable Care Act used the acronym PPACA to refer to the statute. CRS will use "ACA," in conformance with the more widely-used acronym for the law.

[2] For simplicity's sake, the term "plan" is used generically in this report. It applies to different types of health coverage provided to groups (e.g., employees of a single firm) and individuals.

[3] The reference to group markets technically applies to health plans offered by state-licensed insurance carriers and purchased by employers and other plan sponsors. However, health insurance coverage provided through a group may also be sponsored through "self insurance." Groups that self-insure set aside funds to pay for health benefits directly, and those groups bear the risk for covering medical expenses generated by the individuals covered under the self-insured plan. For additional information regarding self-insurance, see CRS Report R41069, *Self-Insured Health Insurance Coverage.*

[4] State regulation of health insurance applies only to state-licensed entities. Since self-insured plans are financed directly by the plan sponsor, such plans are not subject to state law.

(e.g., capital and reserve standards), nature of insurance products (e.g., benefit mandates), and consumer protections (e.g., plan disclosure requirements), among others.

In addition to the state regulation of insurance, the federal government has established federal standards applicable to health coverage and imposes requirements on state-licensed insurance carriers and sponsors of health benefits (e.g., employers). The federal regulation of health coverage is particularly salient with respect to health benefits provided through employment.[5]

ACA follows the model of federalism which has been employed in prior federal reform efforts (e.g., Health Insurance Portability and Accountability Act of 1996). In other words, while ACA establishes many federal rules, the states have primary responsibility for monitoring compliance with and enforcement of such rules. In addition, states may impose additional requirements on insurance carriers and the health plans they offer, provided that the state requirements neither conflict with federal market reforms nor prevent the implementation of such reforms.

ACA Market Reforms

ACA establishes federal requirements that apply to private health insurance. The reforms affect insurance offered to groups and individuals, impose requirements on sponsors of coverage, and, collectively, establish a federal floor with respect to access to coverage, premiums, benefits, cost-sharing, and consumer protections. While such market reforms may be new at the federal level, many of ACA's reforms had already been enacted in some form in some states, with great variation in scope and specificity across the states.

Most of ACA's market reforms become effective in 2014, but a number are already effective.[6] The following sections describe reforms that are effective "immediately" and reforms that are effective for plan years beginning on or after January 1, 2014. The descriptions of the reforms include information from the statute and from regulations, where pertinent. More information about the status of regulations relating to each reform is available in **Appendix A**.

The application of reforms across types of plans is not uniform. Often reforms apply differently to health plans according to the market segment in which the plan is offered and whether the plan has grandfathered status.[7] Moreover, for certain plans the ACA market reforms, as well as other federal health reforms, do not apply. For example, retiree-only health plans are not required to comply with federal health insurance requirements, such as the dependent coverage requirement.[8]

---

[5] Federal regulation applies to both traditional insurance and self-insured plans. For more information about federal regulation of health benefits provided through employment, see CRS Report RS22643, *Regulation of Health Benefits Under ERISA An Outline*.

[6] Most of the private health insurance provisions amend Title XXVII of the Public Health Service Act (PHSA, 42 U.S.C. 300gg et seq.). Title XXVII includes requirements on health insurance coverage for both the group and nongroup markets, enforcement applicable to such requirements, relevant definitions, and other provisions.

[7] A grandfathered health plan refers to an existing plan in which at least one individual has been enrolled since enactment of ACA (March 23, 2010). To maintain grandfathered status, a plan must avoid certain changes to employer contributions, access to coverage, benefits, and cost-sharing (e.g., any increase in co-insurance requirement). For more information about grandfathered status, see CRS Report R41166, *Grandfathered Health Plans Under the Patient Protection and Affordable Care Act (ACA)*.

[8] The federal exemption for retiree-only health plans is not a new exemption. Retiree-only health plans have been exempt from federal health insurance requirements since enactment of the Health Insurance Portability and Accountability Act of 1996. For additional information about these issues, see CRS Report R41166, *Grandfathered* (continued...)

In the text of this report the term "plan" is used generally; for information as to the specific types of plans (i.e., a grandfathered plan in the large group market) to which a reform applies, see **Appendix B**.

"Immediate" Market Reforms

ACA requires implementation of a number of reforms prior to its full implementation date (i.e., prior to plan years beginning on or after January 1, 2014). The ACA term "immediate" refers to the legal effective date of the provision. The actual implementation date, however, may not be immediate due to the time required to make the provision operational.[9]

The following "immediate" reforms are discussed in this section:

- process to review unreasonable rate increases;
- Internet portal to assist consumers in identifying coverage options;
- prohibition on lifetime limits and restriction of annual limits;
- prohibition on rescissions;
- coverage of preventive health services with no cost-sharing;
- extension of dependent coverage;
- prohibition of discrimination based on salary;
- standards related to medical loss ratios and rebates to plan participants;
- appeals process;
- coverage of preexisting health conditions for children;
- patient protections;
- uniform explanation of coverage documents; and
- reporting requirements regarding quality of care.

Process to Review Unreasonable Rate Increases

The Secretary must, in conjunction with the states, establish a process for the annual review of "unreasonable" increases in health insurance rates beginning in the 2010 plan year. Plans are required to submit to the Secretary, and the relevant state, a justification for an unreasonable rate increase prior to implementation.[10]

(...continued)

Health Plans Under the Patient Protection and Affordable Care Act (ACA).

[9] For example, within one year of enactment of ACA, the Secretary of Health and Human Services is required to develop standards for the summary of benefits and coverage (SBC) that plans are expected to provide to their enrollees (§1001: §2715 PHSA). Plans have to begin offering the standardized SBC within two years of enactment.

[10] §1003.

The final rule regarding the review of unreasonable rate increases was published on May 23, 2011.[11] It established a rate review program to ensure that all proposed rate increases in the small group and individual markets that meet or exceed a specified threshold are reviewed by a state or the Centers for Medicare & Medicaid Services (CMS) to determine whether they are unreasonable.[12] Beginning on or after September 1, 2011, a proposed rate increase is tentatively considered unreasonable if the increase either is 10% or more (over a 12-month period beginning on September 1), or meets or exceeds the state-specific threshold.[13] Health plans subject to review are required to submit to the Department of Health and Human Services (HHS) and the relevant state a justification for the proposed rate increase prior to implementation of the premium, and HHS will publicly disclose the information. Note that ACA's rate review process does not establish federal authority to deny implementation of a proposed rate increase. (This is a "sunshine" provision designed to publicly expose rate increases determined to be unreasonable.)[14]

Internet Portal to Assist Consumers in Identifying Coverage Options

The Secretary, in consultation with the states, is required to establish an Internet portal for the public to easily access affordable and comprehensive coverage options. The Secretary is also required to determine the minimum information available through the portal and develop a standardized format for the presentation of information. The interim final rule governing the portal and its content was published on May 5, 2010,[15] and the Internet portal, www.healthcare.gov, was launched on July 1, 2010.[16]

The interim final rule requires the portal to provide, at minimum, information on the following coverage options: health plans offered in the private insurance market; Medicaid and the State Children's Health Insurance Program (CHIP); high risk pools; and small group health plans.

In order to provide coverage information consistently, the interim final rule establishes a standardized format for presentation of information on the portal, including plan eligibility, availability, premium rates, cost-sharing, and the percentage of total premium revenues spent on medical claims compared to administrative costs.

Prohibition of Lifetime Limits and Restriction of Annual Limits

For plan years beginning on or after September 23, 2010, ACA generally prohibits plans from imposing lifetime or "restricted" annual limits on the dollar value of health benefits.[17] The interim final rule on lifetime and annual limits was issued on June 28, 2010.[18]

---

[11] 76 *Federal Register* 29964, May 23, 2011. An amendment to the final rule was published September 6, 2011 (76 *Federal Register* 54969).

[12] ACA does not apply the rate review requirements to grandfathered health plans.

[13] If the a state-specific threshold has not yet been determined by the Secretary, then the threshold for the state is 10%.

[14] For additional information about the final rule related to rate review under ACA, see CRS Congressional Distribution (CD) memorandum "Final Rule related to Rate Review Provision under PPACA," by Bernadette Fernandez and Mark Newsom, August 1, 2011, available upon request.

[15] 75 *Federal Register* 24470, May 5, 2010.

[16] ACA required the Internet portal to become available no later than July 1, 2010. The Department of Health and Human Services launched a Spanish-language version of the site on September 8, 2010.

[17] §1001: §2711 PHSA

The lifetime limits and the restricted annual limits apply specifically to essential health benefits (EHB).[19] The Secretary has not yet issued regulations defining EHB; therefore, the interim final rule states that for plan years beginning before the Secretary defines the EHB, the Departments (the Departments of Health and Human Services, Labor, and Treasury) will take into account good faith efforts to comply with a reasonable interpretation of EHB. For this purpose, a plan must apply the definition of EHB consistently. For example, a plan cannot apply a lifetime limit and a restricted annual limit to the same benefit; applying a lifetime limit implies the benefit is not an EHB, while applying a restricted annual limit implies that the benefit is an EHB. Because the lifetime and annual limit requirements are tied to EHBs, health plans are allowed to impose limits on non-EHBs.

Lifetime Limits

Plans are prohibited from establishing lifetime limits on the dollar value of EHB for any participant or beneficiary. Plans will be permitted to place lifetime limits on specific covered benefits that are not EHB, to the extent that such limits are otherwise permitted by federal and state law.

Under the interim final rule, individuals who reached the lifetime limit under a plan prior to the applicability date of the regulations and are otherwise still eligible under the plan must be provided with a notice that the lifetime limit no longer applies. If these individuals are no longer enrolled in the plan, then the regulations provide an enrollment (or reinstatement in the individual market) opportunity for such individuals. Individuals who are eligible for this enrollment opportunity or reinstatement are allowed to enroll in any of the benefit packages that are available to similarly situated individuals upon initial enrollment. For individuals who reached the lifetime limit under a group health plan offered by an employer, the interim final rule does not specify whether both current and former employees are entitled to the enrollment opportunity.

Restricted Annual Limits

The interim final rule provides that plans may establish a restricted annual limit on the dollar value of EHB prior to January 1, 2014, when annual limits will be prohibited similar to lifetime limits.

The interim final rule adopts a three-year phased in approach for the restricted annual limits. Under these regulations, annual limits on the dollar value of benefits may not be less than the following amounts according to plan years:

- for plan years beginning on or after September 23, 2010, but before September 23, 2011: $750,000;

- for plan years beginning on or after September 23, 2011, but before September 23, 2012: $1.25 million; and

---

(...continued)

[18] 75 *Federal Register* 37188, June 28, 2010.

[19] As defined by §1302(b).

- for plan years beginning on or after September 23, 2012, but before January 1, 2014: $2 million.

Plans may use higher annual limits than the amounts listed above or impose no limits before January 1, 2014. The provision for restricted annual limits sunsets with the plan year beginning January 1, 2014, at which time plans will not be allowed to impose any annual limits.

According to the statute, in defining the restricted annual limits the Secretary should "ensure that access to needed services is made available with a minimal impact on premiums."[20] In the interim final rule it was announced that HHS would establish a process whereby limited benefit plans could request and HHS could grant waivers from the restrictions on annual limits. Limited benefit plans generally offer coverage with restrictive annual limits on total benefits and/or specific service categories. Industry groups that offer limited benefit plans argue that the plans are necessary because more comprehensive coverage is too costly to the workers, and workers would become uninsured without limited benefit plans.[21] Regulators found this argument compelling, and in establishing the waiver process they assumed that applying the restriction on annual limits to limited benefit plans would result in significant decreases in benefits and/or significant increases in premiums.[22]

Prohibition on Rescissions

The practice of "rescission" refers to the retroactive cancellation of medical coverage after an enrollee has become sick or injured. Effective for plan years beginning on or after September 23, 2010, ACA generally prohibits rescissions. Rescissions will still be permitted in cases where the covered individual committed fraud or made an intentional misrepresentation of material fact as prohibited by the terms of the plan. A cancellation of coverage in this case requires prior notice to the enrollee.

The interim final rule on prohibition of rescissions was published on June 28, 2010.[23] The rule requires a health plan to provide at least 30 calendar days advance notice to an individual before coverage may be rescinded. It also clarifies that if any state or federal law that applies to a rescission or cancellation of coverage is more protective of individuals, beyond the standards established by ACA, then that other law would apply.

Coverage of Preventive Health Services with No Cost-Sharing

Effective for plan years beginning on or after September 23, 2010, health plans are required to provide coverage for preventive health services without cost-sharing.[24] The interim final rule for

---

[20] §1001: §2711(a)(2) PHSA

[21] Letter from the National Business Group on Health, to the Secretaries of Health and Human Services, Labor, and the Treasury, August 27, 2010; Letter from the National Restaurant Association, to the Department of Health and Human Services, Office of Consumer Information and Insurance Oversight, August 27, 2010.

[22] For more information about the waiver process for restricted annual limits, see CRS Report R41627, *Waiving the Restriction of Annual Limits in Private Health Insurance* .

[23] 75 *Federal Register* 37188, June 28, 2010.

[24] §1001: §2713 PHSA.

---

the coverage of preventive health services was published on July 19, 2010.[25] The preventive services include the following minimum requirements:

- evidence-based items or services that have in effect a rating of "A" or "B" from the United States Preventive Services Task Force (USPSTF);[26]

- immunizations that have in effect a recommendation from the Advisory Committee on Immunization Practices of the Centers for Disease Control and Prevention (CDC);[27]

- evidence-informed preventive care and screenings (for infants, children, and adolescents) provided for in the comprehensive guidelines supported by the Health Resources and Services Administration (HRSA);[28] and

- additional preventive care and screenings for women not described by the USPSTF, as provided in comprehensive guidelines supported by HRSA.[29]

Additional services not recommended by the USPSTF may be offered, but are not required. For the purposes of this provision and others in federal law, ACA negates the November 2009 USPSTF recommendation that women receive routine screening mammograms beginning at age 50. As a result, plans are required to cover screening mammograms beginning at age 40, based on the prior USPSTF recommendation.[30]

---

[25] 75 *Federal Register* 41726, July 19, 2010. The complete list of recommendations and guidelines required to be covered under the regulations is available at http://www.healthcare.gov/news/factsheets/2010/07/preventive-services-list.html.

[26] The USPSTF is currently sponsored by the Agency for Healthcare Research and Quality (AHRQ), as an independent panel of private-sector experts in prevention and primary care issues. For more background see http://www.ahrq.gov/clinic/uspstfab.htm. A rating of "A" means the preventive service is recommended and there is high certainty that the net benefit is substantial. A rating of "B" means the preventive service is recommended, and there is high certainty that the net benefit is moderate or there is moderate certainty that the net benefit is moderate to substantial. See "U.S. Preventive Services Task Force Grade Definitions" available online at http://www.ahrq.gov/CLINIC/uspstf/gradespost.htm#brec.

[27] The Advisory Committee on Immunization Practices consists of 15 experts in fields associated with immunization who have been selected by the Secretary of Health and Human Services to provide advice and guidance to the Secretary and the CDC on the control of vaccine-preventable diseases. The Committee develops recommendations for the routine administration of vaccines to children and adults in the civilian population; recommendations include age for vaccine administration, number of doses and dosing interval, and precautions and contraindications. http://www.cdc.gov/vaccines/recs/acip/.

[28] HRSA is the primary federal agency within the Department of Health and Human Services for improving access to health care services for people who are uninsured, isolated, or medically vulnerable. HRSA provides leadership and financial support to health care providers in every state and U.S. territory. HRSA grantees provide health care to uninsured people, people living with HIV/AIDS, and pregnant women, mothers and children. For more background see http://www.hrsa.gov/about/default.htm.

[29] HRSA published its guidelines related to women's preventive services in August 2011; the guidelines are found at http://www.hrsa.gov/womensguidelines/. These guidelines include, among other services, coverage for all FDA approved contraceptive methods and sterilization procedures. On February 15, 2012, the Departments of Health and Human Services, Treasury, and Labor (the Departments) issued a final rule that included information regarding the additional preventive care and screenings available to women and their applicability to certain religious employers. On March 21, 2012, the Departments issued an Advance Notice of Proposed Rulemaking with the intention of soliciting comments on proposed amendments to the final rule relating to religious employers and the coverage of contraceptive services. For more information about the requirement to cover contraceptive services without cost sharing, see CRS Report R42370, *Preventive Health Services Regulations Religious Institutions' Objections to Contraceptive Coverage*, by Cynthia Brougher.

[30] For more information about the USPTF recommendation for covering mammograms, see page 32 of CRS Report (continued...)

ACA permits the Secretary to develop guidelines for plans to utilize value-based insurance designs. Value-based insurance designs refer to coverage that encourages the use of services that have clinical benefits exceeding the costs, while discouraging the use of services when the expected clinical benefits do not justify the costs.[31]

The interim final rule clarifies when and how cost-sharing requirements could apply to the recommended preventive services. Among the clarifications, the rule states that with respect to a plan that has a network of providers, the plan is not required to provide coverage for a recommended preventive service that is delivered by an out-of-network provider, and the plan may impose cost-sharing requirements for a recommended preventive service delivered out-of-network. The rule also clarifies that if a recommended preventive service does not specify the frequency, method, treatment, or setting for the service, then the plan can determine coverage limitations by relying on established techniques and relevant evidence.

Extension of Dependent Coverage

Effective for plan years beginning on or after September 23, 2010, ACA requires that if a plan provides for dependent coverage, the plan must make such coverage available to a child under age 26.[32] ACA does not require plans to offer dependent coverage; if a plan chooses not to provide such coverage, nothing in this statute requires them to do so. The age requirement affects only plans that choose to offer dependent coverage.

The interim final rule on the extension of dependent coverage was issued on May 13, 2010,[33] and clarified the following:[34]

- Plans that *offer* dependent coverage must continue to make that offer available until the adult child turns 26 years of age.

- Plans must make coverage available for both married and unmarried adult children under age 26, but not for the adult child's children or spouse.

- With one exception, these provisions apply to grandfathered plans. Prior to 2014, grandfathered group plans are not required to make dependent coverage available to adult children who can enroll in an eligible employer-sponsored plan based on their employment. (However, if a health plan wishes it may voluntarily make dependent coverage available to children with employer offers of coverage.)

(...continued)

R41278, *Public Health, Workforce, Quality, and Related Provisions in PPACA Summary and Timeline*.

[31] Statement of Peter R. Orszag "Health Care and the Budget: Issues and Challenges for Reform" before the Committee on the Budget, United States Senate, June 21, 2007, http://www.cbo.gov/ftpdocs/82xx/doc8255/06-21-HealthCareReform.pdf.

[32] The federal requirements provide a minimum requirement. States that already impose requirements beyond attaining age 26 may continue to do so. To the extent that the state law is more restrictive than the federal law, the federal statute would apply.

[33] 75 *Federal Register* 27122, May 13, 2010.

[34] For more information about the extension of dependent coverage, see CRS Report R41220, *Preexisting Condition Exclusion Provisions for Children and Dependent Coverage under the Patient Protection and Affordable Care Act (ACA)*.

Prohibition of Discrimination Based on Salary

Effective for plan years beginning on or after September 23, 2010, the sponsors of health plans are prohibited from establishing eligibility criteria, for any full-time employee, that are based on the total hourly or annual salary of the employee.[35] In no way will eligibility rules be permitted to discriminate in favor of higher wage employees.

Standards Related to Medical Loss Ratio and Rebates to Plan Participants

Under the ACA, health plans are required to submit to the Secretary a report concerning the percent of premium revenue spent on medical claims ("medical loss ratio" or MLR).[36] The ACA MLR calculation includes adjustments for health quality costs, taxes, regulatory fees, and other factors. The law requires plans in the individual and small group markets to meet a minimum MLR of 80%; for large groups, the minimum MLR is 85%.[37] States are permitted to increase the percentages, and the Secretary may adjust the state percentage for the individual market if it is determined that the application of a minimum MLR of 80% would destabilize the individual market within the state.

These reporting requirements are effective beginning in plan year 2011, with the first annual report due to HHS by June 2012 for the prior plan year. Health plans whose MLR falls below the specified limit must provide rebates to policyholders on a pro rata basis. Any required rebates must be paid to policyholders by August of that year.

The interim final rule relating to the MLR standards was published on December 1, 2010.[38] The interim final rule included explanations of a number of technical issues regarding the calculation and reporting of the MLR, and it provided separate treatment for certain "mini-med" policies for the purpose of the MLR requirements.[39] A final rule published December 7, 2011, modifies certain provisions of the interim final rule, including revising the treatment of mini-med policies.[40]

Appeals Process

Effective for plan years beginning on or after September 23, 2010, the law requires that plans implement an effective appeals process for coverage determinations and claims.[41] The process at a minimum must

---

[35] §1001: §2716 PHSA.

[36] §1001: §2718 PHSA.

[37] Until 2016, ACA allows states to define the small group market as employers who have up to and including 50 employees or up to and including 100 employees; in 2016 the small group market will be defined as employers who have up to and including 100 employees.

[38] 75 *Federal Register* 74864, December 1, 2010.

[39] In the interim final rule it is noted that "mini-med" policies are not defined in statute. Mini-med policies are generally referred to in the interim final rule as policies that often cover health care services similar to the services covered by comprehensive medical plans, but do so with unusually low annual benefit limits, often capping coverage on an annual basis at $5,000 or $10,000.

[40] 76 *Federal Register* 76574, December 7, 2011.

[41] §1001: §2719 PHSA.

- have an internal claims appeals process;

- provide notice to enrollees of available internal and external appeals processes, and the availability of any applicable assistance; and

- allow an enrollee to review their file, present evidence and testimony and to receive continued coverage pending the outcome.

To comply with the requirements for the internal claims appeals process, group plans are expected to initially incorporate the claims and appeals procedures previously established under federal law[42] and will update their processes in accordance with any standards established by the Secretary of Labor. Individual health plans will provide internal claims and appeals procedures set forth under applicable law and updated by the Secretary of HHS.

To comply with the requirements of the external review processes, plans must comply with the applicable state external review process that at a minimum includes the consumer protections set forth in the Uniform External Review Model Act promulgated by the National Association of Insurance Commissioners (NAIC).[43] The health plan is required to implement an effective external review process that meets the minimum standards established by the Secretary of HHS, if the applicable state has not established standards that meet the NAIC model requirements, or if the plan is self-insured and therefore not subject to state insurance regulation.[44]

The interim final rule relating to appeals processes was published on July 23, 2010.[45] The regulations provide updated standards for compliance with the internal claims and appeals processes, and outline a system that explains the applicability to plans of either a state external review process or a federal external review process.

Coverage of Preexisting Health Conditions for Children

ACA prohibits coverage exclusions for children under age 19 with preexisting health conditions, effective for plan years beginning on or after September 23, 2010. In other words, plans may not exclude benefits based on health conditions for qualifying children.

The interim final rule was issued on June 28, 2010, which includes regulations for coverage for preexisting conditions.[46] In the preamble of the rule, it states that this provision "protects individuals under age 19 with a preexisting condition from being denied coverage…based on the preexisting condition."[47] The regulation defines the preexisting conditions exclusion as "a

---

[42] Section 503 of ERISA, codified at 29 CFR §2560.530-1, requires that employee benefit plans provide adequate notice in writing to any participant or beneficiary whose claim for benefits under the plan has been denied, setting forth the specific reasons for such denial, written in a manner calculated to be understood by the participant, and to afford a reasonable opportunity to any participant whose claim for benefits has been denied for a full and fair review by the appropriate named fiduciary of the decision denying the claim.

[43] The NAIC is the organization of insurance regulators for all 50 states, the District of Columbia, and 5 territories. The NAIC is a regulatory support agency that helps state insurance regulators fulfill their obligations to protect the interests of insurance consumers.

[44] State regulation of health insurance applies only to state-licensed entities. Since self-insured plans are financed directly by the plan sponsor, such plans are not subject to state law.

[45] 75 *Federal Register* 43330, July 23, 2010.

[46] 75 *Federal Register* 37188, June 28, 2010.

[47] 75 *Federal Register* 37188, June 28, 2010, p. 37190.

limitation or exclusion of benefits (including a denial of coverage) based on the fact that the condition was present before the effective date of coverage (or if coverage is denied, the date of the denial)." In other words, the rule broadly defined preexisting condition exclusions to include the outright denial of coverage, as well as the exclusion of specific benefits.[48]

Patient Protections

Effective for plan years beginning on or after September 23, 2010, plans are subject to three ACA requirements relating to the choice of health care professionals and one ACA requirement relating to benefits for emergency services.[49] The interim final rule relating to patient protections was published on June 28, 2010.[50]

Regarding the choice of health care professionals, a plan that requires or allows an enrollee to designate a participating primary care provider is required to permit the designation of any participating primary care provider who is available to accept the individual. This same provision applies to pediatric care for any child who is a plan participant. A plan that provides coverage for obstetrical or gynecological care cannot require authorization or referral by the plan or any person (including a primary care provider) for a female enrollee who seeks obstetrical or gynecological care from an in-network health care professional who specializes in obstetrics or gynecology.

If the plan covers services in an emergency department of a hospital, the plan is required to cover those services without the need for any prior authorization and without the imposition of coverage limitations, irrespective of the provider's contractual status with the plan. If the emergency services are provided out-of-network, the cost-sharing requirement will be the same as the cost-sharing for an in-network provider.

Uniform Explanation of Coverage Documents

The ACA required the Secretaries of HHS, Labor, and Treasury (hereinafter, the Secretaries) to develop standards for plans with respect to providing their enrollees with a summary of benefits and coverage (SBC), no later than March 23, 2011.[51] The Secretaries will periodically review and update the standards developed. The Secretaries will consult with the NAIC; representatives of health-insurance related consumer advocacy organizations; health insurance issuers; health care professionals; patient advocates, including those representing individuals with limited English proficiency; and other qualified individuals as deemed appropriate. These federal standards preempt any standards developed under state law. **Table 1** summarizes the standards for the SBC according to the statute.

---

[48] For more information about ACA's prohibition on preexisting condition exclusions for children under 19, see CRS Report R41220, *Preexisting Condition Exclusion Provisions for Children and Dependent Coverage under the Patient Protection and Affordable Care Act (ACA)*.

[49] §1001: §2719A PHSA.

[50] 75 *Federal Register* 37188, June 28, 2010.

[51] §1001: §2715 PHSA. The Secretaries published a notice of proposed rulemaking regarding standards for the disclosure of a summary of benefits and coverage on August 8, 2011 (76 *Federal Register* 52442).

Table 1. Summary of Benefits and Coverage Document Requirements

Issue Area	Requirements
Prohibitions	• Cannot exceed 4 pages in length.
	• Cannot use smaller than 12-point font.
Required description	• Coverage including cost-sharing for each of the essential health benefit categories.
	• Any exceptions, reductions, and limitations on coverage.
	• Renewabi ity and continuation provisions.
	• Whether the plan covers minimum essential benefits.
	• Other benefits as identified by the Secretary.
	• Contact information including a phone number and Internet web address for consumer information.
Other requirements	• Must be presented in a culturally and linguistically appropriate manner utilizing language understandable by the average plan enrollee.
	• Must use uniform definitions of standard insurance and medical terms.
	• Must have a statement ensuring that not less than 60% of allowed costs are covered by the benefits.
	• Must have a statement that the document is a summary and should not be consulted to determine the governing contractual provisions.

Source: CRS analysis of ACA.

The ACA requires that each plan provide a SBC to individuals at the time of application, prior to the time of enrollment or re-enrollment, and when the insurance policy is issued. The SBC can be in paper or electronic form. Enrollees must be given notice of any material changes in benefits no later than 60 days prior to the date that the modifications would become effective. Any entity that willfully fails to provide the information required is subject to a fine of not more than $1,000 for each such failure, defined as each enrollee that did not receive the required information.

The final rule regarding the SBC was published on February 14, 2012.[52] The final rule sets forth standards as to who provides the SBC, to whom, and when. The requirements for the content and appearance of the SBC set forth in the final rule generally mirror the requirements in the statute (presented in **Table 1**). The ACA requires that plans begin providing the SBC no later than March 23, 2012, and the notice of proposed rulemaking (published August 22, 2011)[53] suggests this applicability date. However, after reviewing the comments submitted on this issue, the Secretaries determined that it would not be feasible to require plans to comply with the standards by March 23, 2012. The final rule delays the applicability date of the provision for six months. Generally, plans must comply with the requirements to provide an SBC on or after September 23, 2012.

Reporting Requirements Regarding Quality of Care

Beginning upon ACA enactment (March 23, 2010) and concluding no later than two years after enactment, the Secretary must develop reporting requirements for use by plans, including

---

[52] 77 *Federal Register* 8668, February 14, 2012.

[53] 76 *Federal Register* 52442, August 22, 2011.

regulations governing acceptable provider reimbursement structures.[54] The Secretary must develop these requirements in consultation with experts in health care quality and other stakeholders. Once implemented, plans will annually submit to the Secretary and to enrollees a report addressing whether plan benefits and reimbursement structures do the following:

- improve health outcomes through use of quality reporting, case management, care coordination and chronic disease management;

- implement activities to prevent hospitalization readmissions;

- implement activities to improve patient safety and reduce medical errors through the use of best clinical practices, evidence based medicine, and health information technology; and

- implement wellness and health promotion activities.

The Secretary is required to make these reports available to the public, and is permitted to impose penalties for noncompliance.

Wellness and health promotion activities include personalized wellness and prevention services, and specifically efforts related to smoking cessation, weight management, stress management, physical fitness, nutrition, heart disease prevention, healthy lifestyle support, and diabetes prevention. These services may be made available by entities (for example, health care providers) who conduct health risk assessments or who provide ongoing face-to-face, telephonic, or web-based intervention efforts for program participants.[55]

2014 Market Reforms

In addition to the immediate reforms in ACA, there are additional private insurance market reforms that become effective for plan years beginning on or after January 1, 2014.[56] These reforms include the following:

- nondiscrimination based on health status;

- guaranteed issue and guaranteed renewability;

- coverage of preexisting health conditions (regardless of age);

- nondiscrimination regarding clinical trial participation;

- rating restrictions;

---

[54] §1001: §2717 PHSA. Not later than 180 days after the date on which these regulations are promulgated, the Government Accountability Office (GAO) is required to conduct a study regarding the impact of these activities on the quality and cost of health care, and report its findings to the Senate Committee on Health, Education, Labor, and Pensions, and the House Committee on Energy and Commerce.

[55] With respect to gun rights, a wellness or promotion activity cannot require disclosure or collection of any information in relation to (1) the presence or storage of a lawfully possessed firearm or ammunition in the residence or on the property of an individual, or (2) the lawful use, possession, or storage of a firearm or ammunition by an individual. A health plan issued in accordance with the law is prohibited from increasing premium rates, denying health insurance coverage, and reducing or withholding a discount, rebate, or reward offered for participation in a wellness program on the basis of or on reliance on the lawful ownership, possession, use or storage of a firearm or ammunition.

[56] Unless otherwise noted.

- waiting period limitation; and
- nondiscrimination regarding health care providers.

As in the previous section of this report, it is important to note that the reforms often apply differently to health plans according to the market segment in which the plan is offered and whether the plan has grandfathered status. In the text of this report the term "plan" is used generally; for more specific information as to the specific types of plans (i.e., a grandfathered plan in the large group market) to which the reform applies, see **Appendix B**.

Nondiscrimination Based on Health Status

ACA prohibits health plans from basing eligibility or coverage on health status-related factors.[57] Such factors include health status, medical condition (including both physical and mental illness), claims experience, receipt of health care, medical history, genetic information, evidence of insurability (including conditions arising out of acts of domestic violence), disability, and any other health status-related factor determined appropriate by the Secretary. ACA allows, however, for the offering of premium discounts or rewards based on enrollee participation in wellness programs, in keeping with prior federal law.[58]

Guaranteed Issue and Guaranteed Renewability

ACA requires coverage to be offered on a guaranteed issue basis, as well as on a guaranteed renewal basis.[59] "Guaranteed issue" in health insurance is the requirement that a plan accept every applicant for health coverage, as long as that applicant agrees to the terms and conditions of the insurance offer (such as the premium). "Guaranteed renewability" in health insurance is the requirement on a plan to renew individual coverage at the option of the policyholder, or renew group coverage at the option of the plan sponsor (e.g., employer).

Coverage of Preexisting Health Conditions (Regardless of Age)

Beginning in 2014, ACA prohibits plans from excluding coverage for preexisting health conditions, regardless of the age of the covered individual.[60] A "preexisting health condition" is a medical condition that was present before the date of enrollment for health coverage, whether or not any medical advice, diagnosis, care, or treatment was recommended or received before such date. Excluding coverage for preexisting conditions refers to the circumstance in which an applicant for coverage is offered health insurance but that coverage does not provide benefits for

---

[57] §1201: §2705 PHSA.

[58] The Health Insurance Portability and Accountability Act of 1996 (HIPAA) allows group plans to establish premium discounts or rebates or modify cost-sharing requirements in return for adherence to a wellness program. If a reward is provided based solely on participation in a wellness program, or if it does not provide a reward, the program complies with HIPAA without having to satisfy any additional standards, as long as the program is made available to all similarly situated individuals. If a reward is based on an individual meeting a certain standard relating to a health factor, then the program must meet additional requirements specified in HIPAA regulations. Under ACA, the reward must be capped at 30% of the cost of the employee-only coverage under the plan, but the Secretaries of HHS, Labor, and the Treasury would have the discretion to increase the reward up to 50% of the cost of coverage if the increase is determined to be appropriate.

[59] §1201: §2702, 2703 PHSA.

[60] §1201: §2704 PHSA.

---

treating the applicant's current medical conditions. The interim final rule relating to the coverage of preexisting conditions was issued on June 28, 2010.[61] (For persons under age 19, this provision became effective for plan years beginning on or after September 23, 2010.[62])

Nondiscrimination Regarding Clinical Trial Participation

ACA prohibits health plans from

- prohibiting "qualified individuals" from participating in an approved clinical trial;

- denying, limiting, or placing conditions on the coverage of routine patient costs associated with participation in an approved clinical trial; and

- discriminating against "qualified individuals" on the basis of their participation in approved clinical trials.[63]

ACA defines qualified individual, for purposes of this provision, as an individual who is eligible to participate in an approved clinical trial for treatment of cancer or other life-threatening disease or condition, and who either has a referring health care provider who has concluded that the individual's participation is appropriate, or who provides medical and scientific information establishing that participation in a clinical trial would be appropriate.

Rating Restrictions

ACA imposes adjusted (or modified) community rating rules on the determination of premiums.[64] "Adjusted community rating" rules prohibit health plans from pricing health insurance products based on health factors, but allows it for other key characteristics such as age or gender. ACA's rating rules restrict premium variation to the following factors: self-only or family enrollment; rating area,[65] as specified by the state; age (by no more than a 3 to 1 ratio across age rating bands established by the Secretary, in consultation with the NAIC);[66] and tobacco use (by no more than 1.5 to 1 ratio).[67]

---

[61] 75 *Federal Register* 37188, June 28, 2010.

[62] For additional information about this provision, see CRS Report R41220, *Preexisting Condition Exclusion Provisions for Children and Dependent Coverage under the Patient Protection and Affordable Care Act (ACA)*.

[63] §1201: §2709 PHSA.

[64] §1201: §2701 PHSA.

[65] For example, some states have enacted rating rules in the individual and small group markets that include geography as a characteristic on which premiums may vary. In these cases, the state has established rating areas. Typically, states use counties or zip codes to define those areas.

[66] "By no more than a 3 to 1 ratio" means that a plan will not be allowed to charge an older individual more than 3 times the premium that the plan will charge a younger individual.

[67] "By no more than a 1.5 to 1 ratio" means that a plan will not be allowed to charge a tobacco user more than 1.5 times the premium that the plan will charge an individual who does not use tobacco.

Waiting Period Limitation

ACA prohibits plans from establishing waiting periods greater than 90 days.[68] A "waiting period" refers to the time period that must pass before an individual is eligible to be covered by health benefits.

Nondiscrimination Regarding Health Care Providers

ACA imposes nondiscrimination requirements with respect to health care providers.[69] Plans are not allowed to discriminate, with respect to participation under the plan, against any health care provider who is acting within the scope of that provider's license or certification under applicable state law. This provision does not require a plan to contract with any health care provider willing to abide by the plan's terms and conditions, and the provision cannot be construed as preventing a plan or the Secretary from establishing varying reimbursement rates for providers based on quality or performance measures.

---

[68] §1201: §2708 PHSA.

[69] §1201: §2706 PHSA.

Appendix A. Status of Regulations

Table A-1. Status of Regulations Relating to Health Insurance Market Reforms in ACA, as of September 30, 2011

Health Insurance Market Reform	Status of Federal Regulations	Federal Register Entry	Effective Date of Final or Interim Final Regulations[a]	Applicability and Date[b]
Process to Review Unreasonable Rate Increases	Final rule: May 23, 2011 by the Department of HHS	76 Federal Register 29964	July 18, 2010	No stated applicability
	Amendment to final rule: September 6, 2011 by the Department of HHS	76 Federal Register 54969	November 1, 2011	No stated applicability
Internet Portal to Assist Consumers in Identifying Coverage Options	Interim final rule: May 5, 2010 by the Department of HHS	75 Federal Register 24470	May 10, 2010	No stated applicability
Prohibition of Lifetime Limits and Restriction of Annual Limits	Interim final rule: June 28, 2010 by the Departments of HHS, Labor, and Treasury	75 Federal Register 37188	August 27, 2010	The interim final rule generally applies to group health plans, group health insurance coverage, and individual health insurance coverage, for plan years and policy years beginning on or after September 23, 2010.
Prohibition on Rescissions	Interim final rule: June 28, 2010 by the Departments of HHS, Labor, and Treasury	75 Federal Register 37188	August 27, 2010	The interim final rule generally applies to group health plans, group health insurance coverage, and individual health insurance coverage, for plan years and policy years beginning on or after September 23, 2010.

Health Insurance Market Reform	Status of Federal Regulations	Federal Register Entry	Effective Date of Final or Interim Final Regulations[a]	Applicability and Date[b]
Coverage of Preventive Health Services with No Cost-sharing	Interim final rule: July 19, 2010 by the Departments of HHS, Labor, and Treasury	75 *Federal Register* 41726	September 17, 2010	The interim final rule implements the regulations for coverage of preventive services and generally app ies to group health plans, group health insurance issuers, and individual health insurance issuers for plan years and policy years beginning on or after September 23, 2010.
	Final rule: February 15, 2012 by the Departments of HHS, Labor, and Treasury	77 *Federal Register* 8725	April 16, 2012	The final rule fina izes the provisions of the interim final rule relating to the authorization of an exemption of religious employers from having to cover preventive health services relating to contraception. The final rule generally applies to group health plans and group health insurance issuers beginning April 16, 2012.
	Advance Notice of Proposed Rulemaking (ANPRM): March 21, 2012 by the Departments of HHS, Labor, and Treasury	77 *Federal Register* 16501	No effective date	The ANPRM announces the intention of the Departments to propose amendments to the final rule relating to alternatives for certain religious employers who are required to cover preventive health services relating to contraception. The ANPRM serves as a request for comments, which are due on or before June 19, 2012.
Extension of Dependent Coverage	Interim final rule: May 13, 2010 by the Departments of HHS, Labor, and Treasury	75 *Federal Register* 27122	July 12, 2010	The interim final rule generally app ies to group health plans, group health insurance issuers, and individual health insurance issuers for plan years and policy years beginning on or after September 23, 2010.
Prohibition of Discrimination Based on Salary	No regulatory action to date			
Standards Related to Medical Loss Ratio and Rebates to Plan Participants	Interim final rule: December 1, 2010 by the Department of HHS	75 *Federal Register* 74864	January 1, 2011	The interim final rule generally app ies, beginning January 1, 2011, to health insurance issuers offering group or individual health insurance coverage.
	Final rule: December 7, 2011 by the Department of HHS	76 *Federal Register* 76574	January 3, 2012	The final rule contains amendments to the interim final rule relating to mini-med plans, among other provisions. The amendments in the final rule generally apply to health insurance issuers offering group or individual health insurance coverage beginning January 1, 2012.

Health Insurance Market Reform	Status of Federal Regulations	Federal Register Entry	Effective Date of Final or Interim Final Regulations[a]	Applicability and Date[b]
Appeals Process	Interim final rule: July 23, 2010 by the Departments of HHS, Labor, and Treasury Amendment to interim final rule: June 24, 2011 by the Departments of HHS, Labor, and Treasury	75 *Federal Register* 43330 76 *Federal Register* 37208	September 21, 2010 June 22, 2011	The interim final rule generally applies to group health plans, group health insurance issuers, and individual health insurance issuers for plan years and policy years beginning on or after September 23, 2010.
Coverage of Preexisting Health Conditions for Children	Interim final rule: June 28, 2010 by the Departments of HHS, Labor, and Treasury	75 *Federal Register* 37188	August 27, 2010	The interim final rule generally applies to group health plans, group health insurance coverage, and individual health insurance coverage, for plan years and policy years beginning on or after September 23, 2010.
Patient Protections	Interim final rule: June 28, 2010 by the Departments of HHS, Labor, and Treasury	75 *Federal Register* 37188	August 27, 2010	The interim final rule generally applies to group health plans and group health insurance issuers for plan years beginning on or after September 23, 2010.
Uniform Explanation of Coverage Documents	Final Rule: February 14, 2012 by the Departments of HHS, Labor, and Treasury	77 *Federal Register* 8668	April 16, 2012	The requirements apply to group health plans beginning on the first day of the first open enrollment period that begins on or after September 23, 2012 (for participants who enroll or re-enroll during an open enrollment period) and beginning on the first day of the first plan year that begins on or after September 23, 2012 (for newly eligible individuals). The requirements apply to issuers of coverage in the individual market beginning September 23, 2012.
Reporting Requirements Regarding Quality of Care	No regulatory action to date			
Nondiscrimination Based on Health Status	No regulatory action to date			
Guaranteed Issue and Guaranteed Renewability	No regulatory action to date			

Health Insurance Market Reform	Status of Federal Regulations	Federal Register Entry	Effective Date of Final or Interim Final Regulations[a]	Applicability and Date[b]
Coverage of Preexisting Health Conditions (Regardless of Age)	Interim final regulation: June 28, 2010 by the Departments of HHS, Labor, and Treasury	75 Federal Register 37188	August 27, 2010	The interim final rule generally applies to group health plans, group health insurance coverage, and individual health insurance coverage for plan years and policy years beginning on or after January 1, 2014.
Nondiscrimination Regarding Clinical Trial Participation	No regulatory action to date			
Rating Restrictions	No regulatory action to date			
Waiting Period Limitation	No regulatory action to date			
Nondiscrimination Regarding Health Care Providers	No regulatory action to date			

Source: CRS analysis of federal regulations: 75 Federal Register 24470; 75 Federal Register 27122; 75 Federal Register 37188; 75 Federal Register 41726; 75 Federal Register 43330; 75 Federal Register 74864; 76 Federal Register 29964; 76 Federal Register 37208; 76 Federal Register 46621; 76 Federal Register 52442; 76 Federal Register 54969.

a. The "effective date" of the final or interim final regulation is the date which the regulation takes effect, as stated in the Federal Register notice. The effective date of the regulation is not necessarily the date in which all provisions of the regulation become effective.

b. "Date" in this context is the date on which the regulation generally applies to affected entities, as stated in the Federal Register notice.

Appendix B. Applicability of Market Reforms to Health Plans

Table B-1. Applicability of ACA'S Private Health Insurance Market Reforms to Health Plans

| Provision | Grandfathered Plans[a] | | | New Plans (Non-grandfathered) | | | | |
| | Group Market[b] | | Individual Market[g] | Large Group Market[c] | | Small Group Market[d] | | Individual Market |
	Fully-insured[e]	Self-insured[f]		Fully-insured	Self-insured	Fully-insured	Self-insured	
Process to Review Unreasonable Rate Increases	N.A.	N.A.	N.A.	N.A.[h]	N.A.	yes	N.A.	yes
Prohibition on Lifetime Limits	yes	yes	yes	yes	yes	yes	yes	yes
Restricted Annual Limits	yes	yes	N.A.	yes	yes	yes	yes	yes
Prohibition on Annual Limits	yes	yes	N.A.	yes	yes	yes	yes	yes
Prohibition on Rescissions	yes	yes	yes	yes	yes	yes	yes	yes
Coverage of Preventive Health Services with No Cost-sharing	N.A.	N.A.	N.A.	yes	yes	yes	yes	yes
Extension of Dependent Coverage[i]	yes	yes	yes	yes	yes	yes	yes	yes
Prohibition of Discrimination Based on Salary	N.A.	N.A.	N.A.	yes	N.A.	yes	N.A.	N.A.
Standards Related to Medical Loss Ratio and Rebates to Plan Participants	yes	N.A.	yes	yes	N.A.	yes	N.A.	yes
Appeals Process	N.A.	N.A.	N.A.	yes	yes	yes	yes	yes
Coverage of Preexisting Health Conditions for Children	yes	yes	N.A.	yes	yes	yes	yes	yes
Patient Protections	N.A.	N.A.	N.A.	yes	yes	yes	yes	yes
Uniform Explanation of Coverage Documents	yes	yes	yes	yes	yes	yes	yes	yes
Reporting Requirements Regarding Quality of Care	N.A.	N.A.	N.A.	yes	yes	yes	yes	yes
Nondiscrimination Based on Health Status	N.A.	N.A.	N.A.	yes	yes	yes	yes	yes
Guaranteed Issue & Guaranteed Renewal	N.A.	N.A.	N.A.	yes	N.A.	yes	N.A.	yes

| Provision | Grandfathered Plans[a] | | | New Plans (Non-grandfathered) | | | | |
| | Group Market[b] | | Individual Market[g] | Large Group Market[c] | | Small Group Market[d] | | Individual Market |
	Fully-insured[e]	Self-insured[f]		Fully-insured	Self-insured	Fully-insured	Self-insured	
Coverage of Preexisting Health Conditions (Regardless of Age)	yes	yes	N.A.	yes	yes	yes	yes	yes
Nondiscrimination Regarding Clinical Trial Participation	N.A.	N.A.	N.A.	yes	yes	yes	yes	yes
Rating Restrictions	N.A.	N.A.	N.A.	N.A.	N.A.	yes	N.A.	yes
Waiting Period Limitation	yes	yes	N.A.	yes	yes	yes	yes	N.A.
Nondiscrimination Regarding Health Care Providers	N.A.	N.A.	N.A.	yes	yes	yes	yes	yes

Source: CRS Analysis of ACA.

Notes: N.A. indicates that the reform is not applicable to that type of health insurance plan. These market reforms do not apply to retiree-only health coverage (see footnote 8). The reform "Internet Portal to Assist Consumers in Identifying Coverage Options" is not included in this table because the reform does not apply to health plans.

a. A grandfathered plan refers to an existing group health plan or a health insurance plan/policy in which at least one individual is enrolled since March 23, 2010. To maintain grandfathered status, a plan must avoid certain changes to benefits, cost-sharing, employer contributions, and access to coverage.

b. Health insurance can be provided to a group of people that are drawn together by an employer or other organization, such as a trade union. Such groups are generally formed for some purpose other than obtaining insurance, like employment. When insurance is provided to a group, it is referred to as "group coverage" or "group insurance." In the group market, the entity that purchases health insurance on behalf of a group is referred to as the plan "sponsor."

c. Prior to ACA, large groups were defined as groups with more than 50 workers. For plan years beginning before January 1, 2016, a state may elect to keep the previous definition of large groups, or change the definition to include those groups with more than 100 workers, applicable to ACA-created exchanges and market reforms. For plan years beginning on or after January 1, 2016, large groups must be defined as groups with more than 100 workers.

d. Prior to ACA, small groups were defined as groups with 2 to 50 workers, although some states also included self-employed individuals ("groups of one") in the small group market. For plan years beginning before January 1, 2016, a state may elect to keep the previous definition of small groups, or change the definition to include those groups with 1-100 workers, applicable to ACA-created exchanges and market reforms. For plan years beginning on or after January 1, 2016, small groups must be defined as groups with 1-100 workers.

e. A fully-insured health plan is one in which the plan sponsor purchases health coverage from a state-licensed insurance carrier; the carrier assumes the risk of paying the medical claims of the sponsor's enrolled members.

f. Self-insured plans refer to health coverage that is provided directly by the organization seeking coverage for its members (e.g. a firm providing health benefits to its employees). Such organizations set aside funds and pay for health benefits directly. Under self insurance, the organization bears the risk for covering medical claims.

g. Consumers who are not associated with a group can obtain health coverage by purchasing it directly from an insurance carrier in the individual (or nongroup) health insurance market.

h. The final rule regarding rate review specified that this provision would apply only to nongroup and fully-insured, small group coverage, and not to large groups.

i. Prior to 2014, grandfathered group health plans are not required to make dependent coverage available to adult children who can enroll in an eligible employer-sponsored health plan based on their employment; however, if a plan wishes to make dependent coverage available to such adult children it may voluntarily do so.

Author Contact Information

Annie L. Mach
Analyst in Health Care Financing
amach@crs.loc.gov, 7-7825

Bernadette Fernandez
Specialist in Health Care Financing
bfernandez@crs.loc.gov, 7-0322

www.ingramcontent.com/pod-product-compliance
Lightning Source LLC
Chambersburg PA
CBHW081416170526
45166CB00010B/3362